FACILITATOR GUIDE for

FIFTH EDITION

Anatomy of WRITING FOR PUBLICATION FOR NURSES

CYNTHIA SAVER, MS, RN

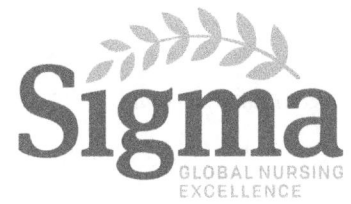

Copyright © 2024 by Cynthia Saver

All rights reserved. This book is protected by copyright. No part of it may be reproduced, stored in a retrieval system, or transmitted in any form or by any means, electronic, mechanical, photocopying, recording, or otherwise, without written permission from the publisher. Any trademarks, service marks, design rights, or similar rights that are mentioned, used, or cited in this book are the property of their respective owners. Their use here does not imply that you may use them for a similar or any other purpose.

This book is not intended to be a substitute for the medical advice of a licensed medical professional. The author and publisher have made every effort to ensure the accuracy of the information contained within at the time of its publication and shall have no liability or responsibility to any person or entity regarding any loss or damage incurred, or alleged to have incurred, directly or indirectly, by the information contained in this book. The author and publisher make no warranties, express or implied, with respect to its content, and no warranties may be created or extended by sales representatives or written sales materials. The author and publisher have no responsibility for the consistency or accuracy of URLs and content of third-party websites referenced in this book.

Sigma Theta Tau International Honor Society of Nursing (Sigma) is a nonprofit organization whose mission is developing nurse leaders anywhere to improve healthcare everywhere. Founded in 1922, Sigma has more than 135,000 active members in over 100 countries and territories. Members include practicing nurses, instructors, researchers, policymakers, entrepreneurs, and others. Sigma's more than 540 chapters are located at more than 700 institutions of higher education throughout Armenia, Australia, Botswana, Brazil, Canada, Chile, Colombia, Croatia, England, Eswatini, Finland, Ghana, Hong Kong, Ireland, Israel, Italy, Jamaica, Japan, Jordan, Kenya, Lebanon, Malawi, Mexico, the Netherlands, Nigeria, Pakistan, Philippines, Portugal, Puerto Rico, Scotland, Singapore, South Africa, South Korea, Sweden, Taiwan, Tanzania, Thailand, the United States, and Wales. Learn more at www.sigmanursing.org.

Sigma Theta Tau International
550 West North Street
Indianapolis, IN, USA 46202

To request a review copy for course adoption, order additional books, buy in bulk, or purchase for corporate use, contact Sigma Marketplace at 888.654.4968 (US/Canada toll-free), +1.317.687.2256 (International), or solutions@sigmamarketplace.org.

To request author information, or for speaker or other media requests, contact Sigma Marketing at 888.634.7575 (US/Canada toll-free) or +1.317.634.8171 (International).

PRINT ISBN: 9781646481651
EPUB ISBN: 9781646481668
PDF ISBN: 9781646481675

Publisher: Dustin Sullivan
Managing Editor: Carla Hall
Acquisitions Editor: Emily Hatch
Publications Specialist: Todd Lothery
Development Editor: Jillmarie Leeper Sycamore
Project Editor: Jillmarie Leeper Sycamore
Cover Designer: Rebecca Batchelor
Copy Editor: Erin Geile
Interior Design/Page Layout: Kim Scott/Bumpy Design
Proofreader: Todd Lothery

To all my writing mentors over the years, my family (especially my mother, who introduced me to the pleasure of reading and writing), and Jackie, Terry, and David.

Acknowledgments

Thank you to my incredible team of contributors, most of whom have been with me through all five editions of this book. I am honored to be in such stellar company. The contributors bring a wonderful wealth of collective knowledge that reflects all the roles of publishing—author, editor, peer reviewer, designer, publisher—along with a strong commitment to help nurses share their expertise through publishing. I truly appreciate how they have generously shared their talents. I also appreciate the many others who read portions of the book and gave valuable feedback.

Thanks to Joan Borgatti for first linking anatomy to writing and to Patricia Dwyer Schull for her insightful comments and unfailing support.

Special thanks to the talented staff members at Sigma Theta Tau International, who always make authors look great: to Jill Sycamore and Erin Geile for their expert editing; Todd Lothery for proofreading; and Kim Scott for design and layout.

Publishing is truly a team effort!

About the Editor and Lead Author

Cynthia Saver, MS, RN, of CLS Development, is an award-winning author. She has more than five decades of experience in nursing, including more than four decades of publishing experience as a writer, editor, and senior vice president of editorial teams. Saver has written for many nursing publications, including *American Nurse Journal, American Journal of Nursing, AORN Journal, Journal of Nursing Regulation, Nurse Leader, Nursing Management, Nursing Spectrum, The Nurse Practitioner,* and *OR Manager,* to name a few. Her writing experience includes a 10-part writing for publication series for *AORN Journal,* research reports, case studies, interviews, clinical articles, and continuing education programs. She has written materials for nurses, physicians, pharmacists, social workers, physical therapists, occupational therapists, dentists, and other healthcare professionals.

Saver has worked with the top publishers as an author, editor, managing editor, and editorial director, including Editorial Director for *American Nurse Journal,* the official journal of the American Nurses Association, and Executive Vice President of Editorial for *Nursing Spectrum.* She was an invited reviewer for the *Publication Manual of the American Psychological Association* (7th ed., 2020). Saver's writing for publication program for nurses has received excellent reviews, and participants have published many articles. She received her master's degree in nursing from The Ohio State University, is an author-in-residence for *Nurse Author & Editor,* serves on the editorial board for *The Maryland Nurse,* and blogs for *American Nurse Journal* at The Writing Mind (https://www.myamericannurse.com/category/the-writing-mind).

About the Contributing Authors

Mary Alexander, MA, RN, CRNI, CAE, FAAN, is Chief Executive Officer Emerita at the Infusion Society (INS). She was named CEO of the INS and the Infusion Nurses Certification Corporation (INCC) in 1997 and served until her retirement in 2023. For 25 years as Editor of the *Journal of Infusion Nursing,* Alexander wrote bimonthly columns and had editorial responsibilities for *INSider,* the bimonthly membership newsletter. She is Editor of *Core Curriculum for Infusion Nursing* (5th ed.) and Editor-in-Chief of the INS textbook *Infusion Nursing: An Evidence-Based Approach.* Alexander's areas of expertise include infusion therapy with an emphasis on patient safety, practitioner competency, and standards development. Her clinical experience spans a variety of practice settings, including home care, alternative sites, and acute care settings.

Nancy J. Brent, JD, MS, RN, is a nurse attorney in private law practice. After practicing and teaching psychiatric nursing for more than 15 years, Brent graduated from Loyola University of Chicago School of Law in 1981. Her private practice is concentrated in professional licensure defense for nurses and other healthcare providers, consultation to nurses and school of nursing faculty, and educational programs in law and nursing practice for nurses and other healthcare groups. She has published extensively in the area of law and nursing practice. Brent is also the author of a legal blog at Nurse.com (https://www.nurse.com/blog/author/nbrent).

Christopher Burton, DPhil, RN, is Professor of Health Services Research, Health Foundation Improvement Science Fellow, Canterbury Christ Church University, Canterbury, Kent, England. Burton is a registered nurse with a special interest in supporting patients affected by stroke and long-term health conditions. As Professor of Health Services Research at Canterbury Christ Church University, he leads a programme of research and scholarship that seeks to close the gap between evidence, policy, and practice. He works with researchers across the globe to develop knowledge of "what works" in implementation and improvement and networks to embed this within educational programmes for nurses and other healthcare professionals.

Marianne Ditomassi, DNP, MBA, RN, NEA-BC, FAAN, is Executive Director of Nursing and Patient Care Services Operations and Magnet® Recognition at Massachusetts General Hospital (MGH). Ditomassi is the Chief of Staff for the Senior Vice President for Patient Care and Chief Nurse, who oversees the operations of nursing, therapy departments, and social services. Ditomassi's key areas of accountability include strategic planning, professional practice environment development and evaluation, recruitment and retention initiatives, business planning, fundraising, and communications. She also is the Magnet Program Director for MGH and coordinated MGH's initial Magnet designation journey in 2003 and subsequent Magnet redesignations in 2008, 2013, 2018, and 2023.

Susan Gennaro, PhD, RN, FAAN, is a Professor in the Connell School of Nursing at Boston College. She is an internationally renowned perinatal clinician and scholar whose research has improved healthcare for childbearing women and their families around the world. She is also the Editor of the *Journal of Nursing Scholarship*, which is read in more than 103 countries and whose mission is to advance knowledge to improve the health of the world's people. Gennaro has been active in supporting that mission by leading an understanding of how best to promote global dissemination of nursing scholarship.

Pamela J. Haylock, PhD, RN, FAAN, is a nurse educator and cancer survivorship consultant. Throughout her career, Haylock has held staff, advanced practice, management, nursing education, and consultation roles and is a past President of the Oncology Nursing Society. She contributes to professional and peer-reviewed literature as an author, editor, and manuscript reviewer, and by serving on professional journals' editorial boards. Her introduction to writing for general audiences was as coauthor of *Women's Cancers: How to Prevent Them, How to Treat Them, How to Beat Them* (with Kerry A. McGinn), followed by *Cancer Doesn't Have to Hurt* (with coauthor Carol P. Curtiss), and as editor and contributor for *Men's Cancers: How to Prevent Them, How to Treat Them, How to Beat Them*. Haylock was a team member and writer for the National Coalition for Cancer Survivorship's award-winning *Cancer Survival Toolbox*—audio instructional programs for survivors and family caregivers. In 2002, Haylock received the Distinguished Alumni Award for Service from the University of Iowa College of Nursing, and in 2008, she received a Distinguished Alumni Award for Service from the University of Iowa. She was inducted as a Fellow of the American Academy of Nursing in 2011.

Lisa Hopp, PhD, RN, FAAN, is Dean Emerita, Nursing, Purdue University Northwest; and Vice Dean, College of Nursing, Rosalind Franklin University of Medicine and Science, Chicago. She is internationally recognized for her work in evidence-based nursing practice. She has trained hundreds of faculty, advanced practice nurses, and library scientists in systematic review methodologies. Hopp is the founding director of the Indiana Center for Evidence Based Nursing, part of a global collaboration of JBI (formerly Joanna Briggs Institute) centers and groups that aim to improve healthcare outcomes through evidence-based healthcare. She continues to serve as a Deputy Director for a JBI Center of Excellence at Rosalind Franklin University of Medicine and

Science. She has been an educator for more than 30 years, helping prepare future advanced practice and registered nurses.

Timothy Landers, PhD, RN, APRN-CNP, CIC, FAAN, is a nurse practitioner and infection prevention researcher. His research focuses on practical, evidence-based infection prevention strategies to address the most pressing problems in infectious disease prevention. He has written multiple guidelines on infection prevention using a One Health paradigm. Landers was an Associate Professor at The Ohio State University for 10 years, where he taught in the graduate programs, and has served as the Nurse Scientist at Nationwide Children's Hospital. He was a Fulbright Scholar in Ethiopia from 2017 to 2018. Landers was on the editorial board of the *American Journal of Infection Control*, and his scholarly work has been widely featured in the media and lay press. He has mentored students and nurses in writing and publishing for many years.

Fidelindo Lim, DNP, CCRN, FAAN, is a Clinical Associate Professor in the NYU Rory Meyers College of Nursing at New York University. He has worked as a critical care nurse for 18 years, and concurrently, since 1996, as a nursing faculty member. Lim has published more than 200 articles on an array of topics, including clinical practice, geriatrics, nursing education, LGBTQ+ health, reflective practice, preceptorship, men in nursing, nursing humanities, and Florence Nightingale. *American Nurse Journal,* the official journal of the American Nurses Association, designated him as a Nurse Influencer. Lim is a Fellow of the American Academy of Nursing. He holds a DNP from Northeastern University, a master of arts in nursing education from NYU, and a BSN from Far Eastern University in Manila, Philippines.

Deborah Lindell, DNP, MSN, RN, CNE, ANEF, FAAN, is a Professor in the Frances Payne Bolton School of Nursing at Case Western Reserve University, Cleveland, Ohio. For over 30 years, Lindell has been an educator and administrator in undergraduate and graduate nursing programs. Currently, she coordinates Frances Payne Bolton School of Nursing's schoolwide Curriculum Transformation Initiative. Lindell's clinical background is in community/public health nursing, and her scholarship concerns nursing theory, history, and education. Internationally, she has consulted and taught masters' level courses in Vietnam and China and was a Fulbright Scholar in Kenya from 2021 to 2022. Lindell was instrumental in the development and implementation of the National League for Nursing's Certified Nurse Educator (CNE) Program and served as Chair of the CNE Commission. She is a Fellow in the NLN's Academy of Nursing Education and in the American Academy of Nursing.

Kayla Little, MSN, APRN, AGCNS-BC, PCCN, is a Clinical Nurse Specialist who supports the cardiovascular medicine, heart and lung transplant, and vascular surgery stepdown nursing units within the Heart, Vascular, and Thoracic Institute at the Cleveland Clinic Main Campus. She earned a BSN from Walsh University and an MSN from Kent State University. Little has been published in *Critical Care Nurse Journal, American Nurse Journal,* and *Clinical Nurse Specialist Journal*. She was an invited reviewer for the *AACN Procedure Manual for Progressive and Critical Care* (8th ed., 2023) and a contributor to *Foundations of Clinical Nurse Specialist Practice* (4th ed.). Little was the recipient of the Rising Star Clinical Nurse Specialist of the Year Award in 2022 from the National Association of Clinical Nurse Specialists. Her passion for mentoring nurses and future Clinical Nurse Specialists led her to be the recipient of the Barbara Donaho Distinguished Leadership in Learning Award from Kent State University in 2023. Little values lifelong learning and professional citizenship. She is a column editor for the *Clinical Nurse Specialist Journal* and serves on the board of directors for the National Association of Clinical Nurse Specialists.

Tina M. Marrelli, MSN, MA, RN, FAAN, is President of Marrelli and Associates Inc., a consulting and publishing firm. She is the author of 13 best-selling and award-winning healthcare books, including *Handbook of Home Health Standards: Quality, Documentation, and Reimbursement* (6th ed.); *Nurse Manager's Survival Guide* (4th ed.); *Hospice & Palliative Care Handbook* (4th ed.); *Home Health Aide: Guidelines for Care – Instructor Manual* (3rd ed.); and *A Guide for Caregiving: What's Next? Planning for Safety, Quality, and Compassionate Care for Your Loved One and Yourself*. Marrelli has also authored apps to assist with care planning. She received her BSN degree from Duke University and has master's degrees in health administration and in nursing. Marrelli has worked at CMS on Medicare home care and hospice Part A policy and operations, been the editor of three peer-reviewed publications, and practiced as a visiting nurse and manager in home care and hospice.

Cheryl L. Mee, MSN, MBA, RN, FAAN, leads the editorial team for *American Nurse Journal*, the official journal of the American Nurses Association. She is an Adjunct Instructor at Frances Payne Bolton School of Nursing, Case Western Reserve University, Cleveland, Ohio, working with doctor of nursing practice students. Her past roles include Editor-in-Chief for *Nursing* and Vice President of Nursing and Health Professions Journals at Elsevier. Mee has written over 130 articles addressing the current, persistent, challenging problems confronting nurses delivering direct patient care. She is on the board of Americans for Native Americans, where she has worked to provide scholarships, NCLEX fees, and varied clinical experiences for Native American nursing students, as well as planning annual health screening programs assessing hundreds of Navajo elementary school children.

Patricia Gonce Morton, PhD, RN, ACNP-BC, FAAN, is Dean Emeritus, University of Utah College of Nursing, where she served as Dean and Professor and held the Louis Peery Endowed Presidential Chair. Before her deanship, Morton served in various administrative positions at the University of Maryland School of Nursing. An educator and scholar who is known for her work in critical care nursing and nursing education, Morton has written multiple editions of three textbooks, numerous book chapters, and over 60 journal articles. She has served on the editorial board of eight nursing journals and for seven years was the Editor of the journal *AACN Clinical Issues: Advanced Practice in Acute and Critical Care*, sponsored by the American Association of Critical-Care Nurses. Currently, Morton is Editor of the *Journal of Professional Nursing*, sponsored by the American Association of Colleges of Nursing. She also is an author-in-residence for *Nurse Author & Editor*. In recognition of her contributions to nursing and healthcare, Morton was inducted as a Fellow in the American Academy of Nursing in 1999.

Cindy L. Munro, PhD, RN, ANP-BC, FAAN, FAANP, is Dean and Professor at the University of Miami School of Nursing and Health Studies in Coral Gables, Florida. She has served as Coeditor of *American Journal of Critical Care* for more than 10 years. An experienced peer reviewer, she has published more than 200 articles and presented at many national and international conferences. Munro received a diploma from York Hospital School of Nursing, a BSN from Millersville University of Pennsylvania, and an MSN from the University of Delaware. She earned her PhD in nursing and microbiology and immunology at Virginia Commonwealth University. Her NIH-funded research on oral care in critically ill adults has had an important effect on clinical practice. In 2016, Sigma Theta Tau International Honor Society of Nursing inducted Munro into its International Nurse Researcher Hall of Fame. She is an American Academy of Nursing Edge Runner.

Sandra M. Nettina, MSN, ANP-BC, is owner and founder of Prime Care House Calls in West Friendship, Maryland, and Editor of *The Lippincott Manual of Nursing Practice*. She attended the Sisters of Charity Hospital School of Nursing in Buffalo, New York; completed a bachelor's degree at Marymount College of Virginia; and received her MSN from the University of Pennsylvania, Philadelphia. As an adult nurse practitioner, Nettina's multidimensional career includes founding a nurse practitioner independent-house-calls practice; writing, editing, and reviewing for several publishing companies; providing leadership in her state nurse practitioner association; and volunteering for several health-related organizations.

Leslie H. Nicoll, PhD, MBA, RN, FAAN, is principal and owner of Maine Desk LLC and Editor-in-Chief of *CIN: Computers, Informatics, Nursing*. Nicoll has more than 43 years of experience in nursing and healthcare and has worked in clinical practice, research, and academia. She founded her own business, Maine Desk LLC, in 2001. Nicoll has been the Editor-in-Chief of *CIN: Computers, Informatics, Nursing* since 1995 and was the Editor-in-Chief of *Nurse Author & Editor* from 2014 to 2022. She served as Editor-in-Chief of *The Journal of Hospice and Palliative Nursing* for eight years (2001–2009). Nicoll is the author of more than 130 published professional articles, book chapters, and books, including *Writing in the Digital Age: Savvy Publishing for Healthcare Professionals*, coauthored with Peggy L. Chinn, and *The Editor's Handbook* (3rd ed.). She was the founding editor of *Perspectives on Nursing Theory*. In the non-nursing literature, she is the author of four "For Dummies" books, including *Kindle Paperwhite For Dummies*. Nicoll enjoys helping nurses and other healthcare professionals achieve their publication goals. She has done this through one-on-one support in her business as well as leading writing workshops for the National League for Nursing, a consortium of universities in Switzerland, and various colleges and schools of nursing in the United States. Nicoll became a Fellow in the American Academy of Nursing in 2014. She is active in INANE: The International Academy of Nursing Editors and received their leadership award for excellence in editorial publication in 2015.

Susanne J. Pavlovich-Danis, MSN, RN, APRN-C, CDCES, is Director of Clinical Continuing Education at TeamHealth Institute in Knoxville, Tennessee. She has 42 years of experience in nursing and healthcare in diverse clinical, academic, and consultant-based settings. As Director of Clinical Continuing Education at TeamHealth Institute, she currently oversees the Joint Accreditation for Interprofessional Continuing Education that includes the Accreditation Council for Continuing Medical Education (ACCME), the Accreditation Council for Pharmacy Education (ACPE), and the American Nurses Credentialing Center (ANCC). She serves in the chief editorial capacity for more than 600 annual continuing education activities nationwide for a multidisciplinary audience. She also maintains a private adult primary care practice in Plantation, Florida, and is a certified diabetes care and education specialist (CDCES). Pavlovich-Danis is an approved continuing nursing education provider for the Florida Board of Nursing. She has been published in the nursing literature more than 500 times since 1996 and lectured nationally and internationally.

Demetrius J. Porche, DNS, PhD, PCC, ANEF, FACHE, FAANP, FAAN, is Dean and Professor at the Louisiana State University Health Sciences Center School of Nursing in New Orleans. Porche is Chief Editor of the *American Journal of Men's Health* and was Associate Editor of the *Journal of the Association of Nurses in AIDS* for 10 years. He is a Virginia Henderson Fellow of Sigma Theta Tau International and a Society of Luther Christman Fellow for Contributions to Nursing by Men. He is also a Fellow in the National League for Nursing Nurse Educator Academy, the American

Academy of Nursing, and the American Academy of Nurse Practitioners. He is board-certified in healthcare by the American College of Healthcare Executives. Porche is author of *Health Policy: Application for Nurses and Other Health Care Professionals* (2nd ed.) and *Epidemiology for the Advanced Practice Nurse: A Population Health Approach*. He has published many articles in peer-reviewed journals.

Jo Rycroft-Malone, OBE, PhD, MSc, BSc (Hons), RN, is Distinguished Professor, Executive Dean of Health & Medicine at Lancaster University, England. She has a nursing background and is a health services researcher who studies the processes and outcomes of evidence-informed service delivery in different health service contexts across the globe. Rycroft-Malone is also the Director of the National Institute for Health Research (NIHR) Health Services & Delivery Research Programme, which funds research to generate evidence to improve the quality, accessibility, and organisation of health and care services in the United Kingdom. She was the inaugural Editor of *Worldviews on Evidence-Based Nursing*.

Nadine Salmon, MSN, RN, NPD-BC, IBCLC, is a Curriculum Designer in the Acute Vertical at Relias, a leading provider of online continuing education for healthcare, senior care, and disability professionals. Salmon obtained her BSN in South Africa more than 30 years ago and has worked as an RN in South Africa, England, and the United States in various settings, including labor and delivery, postpartum, home health, and adult surgical units. She has an MSN with an emphasis in leadership in healthcare systems from Grand Canyon University. Salmon has served as an appraiser for the American Nurses Credentialing Center, is certified in nursing professional development, and is an international board-certified lactation consultant. She has been involved in creating nursing continuing education content and certification review courses for more than 20 years, and enjoys collaborating with subject matter expert writers, instructional designers, and quality assurance and education technicians in developing continuing education courses for nurses, physicians, and allied health professionals.

Patricia Dwyer Schull, MSN, BS, is President of MedVantage Publishing LLC. She has more than 30 years' experience in medical and nursing publishing. She has published, written, and edited many nursing journals, books, websites, and other healthcare publications. Her company offers publishing solutions that support and educate healthcare professionals, including developing and launching the award-winning publications *Nursing Spectrum and McGraw Hill Nurses Drug Handbook*, *American Nurse Journal* (official journal of the American Nurses Association), and *Journal of Nursing Regulation* (official journal of the National Council of State Boards of Nursing). Previously, Schull held executive management positions with Reed Elsevier (Springhouse Corporation) and Wolters Kluwer (Lippincott, Williams & Wilkins), where she was responsible for leading editorial, sales, marketing, and new product development of nursing publications. Before entering the publishing industry, she practiced as a registered nurse in direct patient care, hospital management, and staff education.

Stephanie J. Schulte, MLIS, is Professor, Assistant Vice President, Health Sciences, and Director, Health Sciences Library at The Ohio State University. She is a library director and faculty health sciences librarian who specializes in teaching students, faculty, and staff advanced skills to support evidence-based practice and research endeavors. Her research work currently focuses on librarians who work directly with basic or life scientists. Schulte teaches within the medical school curriculum as well as the biomedical sciences undergraduate program at The Ohio State University and leads a team of research and education librarians serving five health sciences colleges and a large academic medical center. She has been active in university governance, the Medical Library Association, and the Midwest Chapter of the Medical Library Association.

Rose O. Sherman, EdD, RN, NEA-BC, FAAN, is Emeritus Professor, Christine E. Lynn College of Nursing at Florida Atlantic University, and a faculty member of the Marian K. Shaughnessy Nursing Leadership Academy at Case Western Reserve University. Before becoming a faculty member, Sherman was a nurse leader with the Department of Veterans Affairs for 25 years. She edits a popular leadership blog (www.emergingrnleader.com) and is Editor-in-Chief of *Nurse Leader*, the official journal of the American Organization for Nursing Leadership. Sherman has extensive experience with both podium and poster presentations at professional conferences. She has also served as an abstract reviewer for numerous professional conferences at the state and national levels. Sherman is a Gallup-certified strengths coach and author of the books *The Nurse Leader Coach: Become the Boss No One Wants to Leave*, *The Nuts and Bolts of Nursing Leadership: Your Toolkit for Success*, and *A Team Approach to Nursing Care Delivery: Tactics for Working Better Together.*

Lorraine Steefel, DNP, RN, CTN-A, is Director of LTS Writing/Mentoring & Editorial Services for RNs and students. She is a professional writer and writing consultant who has presented webinars and writing for publication workshops to nurses across the country. Her experience includes teaching academic writing to all levels of nursing students, especially mentoring DNP students who are writing their capstone project papers and turning them into published articles. Steefel has been widely published in peer-reviewed journals, nursing magazines, and on websites. She served as the American Nurses Association representative to the Centers for Disease Control and Prevention (CDC) Work Group to update the CDC website on ME/CFS (myalgic encephalomyelitis/chronic fatigue syndrome). Her book *What Nurses Know...Chronic Fatigue Syndrome* was published by Demos Publishers in New York. Steefel is a member of the Research Roadmap for ME/CFS for the National Institutes of Health, which is creating webinars about the illness to identify research priorities to move the field forward. Steefel is the Associate Editor for Peer Review for *Creative Nursing: A Journal of Values, Issues, Experience & Collaboration*, published by Sage, and an editorial board member of the *Journal of Nursing Practice, Applications and Reviews of Research* (JNPARR), the official journal of the Philippine Nurses Association of America. She is a mentor for the Thomas Edison State University School of Nursing online nursing program.

Table of Contents

About the Editor and Lead Author v
About the Contributing Authors v
Introduction to the Facilitator Guide xiii

Part I: A Primer on Writing and Publishing 1

1. Anatomy of Writing 2
   Cynthia Saver

2. Finding, Refining, and Defining a Topic 3
   Patricia Dwyer Schull and Cynthia Saver

3. How to Select and Query a Publication 4
   Cynthia Saver

4. Finding and Documenting Sources 6
   Leslie H. Nicoll

5. Organizing the Article 8
   Kayla Little and Mary Alexander

6. Writing Skills Lab 9
   Cynthia Saver

7. All About Graphics 11
   Susanne J. Pavlovich-Danis

8. Submissions and Revisions 13
   Patricia Gonce Morton and Tina M. Marrelli

9. Writing a Peer Review 14
   Cindy L. Munro

10. Publishing for Global Authors 16
    Susan Gennaro

11. Legal and Ethical Issues 17
    Nancy J. Brent

12. Promoting Your Work 18
    Timothy Landers and Stephanie J. Schulte

Part II: Tips for Writing Different Types of Articles 21

13. Writing the Clinical Article 22
    Cheryl L. Mee and Fidelindo Lim

14. Writing the Research Report 23
    Patricia Gonce Morton

15. Writing the Review Article 24
    Lisa Hopp

16. Reporting the Quality Improvement or Evidence-Based Practice Project 25
    Jo Rycroft-Malone and Christopher Burton

17. Writing for Presentations 27
    Rose O. Sherman

18. From Student Project or Dissertation to Publication 28
    Deborah Lindell and Lorraine Steefel

19. Writing a Continuing Professional Development Activity 29
    Nadine Salmon

20. Writing the Nursing Narrative 30
    Marianne Ditomassi

21. Think Outside the Journal: Alternative Publication Options 32
    Demetrius J. Porche

22. Writing a Book or Book Chapter 33
    Sandra M. Nettina

23. Writing for a General Audience 34
    Pamela J. Haylock

Introduction to the Facilitator Guide

Anatomy of Writing for Publication, Fifth Edition, is designed to take the mystery out of writing by providing practical advice from a wealth of experts in the publishing field. Not only have these experts written published articles of their own, but many have also sat on the other side of the table in the publishing world, editing manuscripts and making decisions as to what gets published, so each offers a unique and valuable perspective. The book walks readers through the writing process, with in-depth tips, examples, and resources to provide stepping stones along the way. The ultimate goal is to get nurses and students writing!

The book is divided into two parts.

Part I, "A Primer on Writing and Publishing," describes the basics of publishing, from generating a great idea and writing an article to revising a manuscript and seeing it published. The goal is to give readers a solid understanding of the publishing process. Chapters 1–8 serve as a primer—when followed in order, students can use these chapters as a guide to create a finished article, from idea conception to submitting a manuscript. Students also should consider the information in Chapter 11, "Legal and Ethical Issues."

Part II, "Tips for Writing Different Types of Articles," is where students can apply what they learned in Part I to a variety of content styles. It isn't necessary to have the students read these chapters sequentially—rather, you can pick and choose which areas best fit the goals of the class. For example, graduate students might be particularly interested in Chapter 18, "From Student Project or Dissertation to Publication." Undergraduate students might benefit more from Chapter 13, "Writing the Clinical Article." Chapters not covered in class can be resources for future writing projects.

Each chapter contains these elements:

- **Opening quotes:** Quotes at the start of each chapter provide pithy words of wisdom related to the craft of writing.
- **What You'll Learn in This Chapter:** This provides an overview of what's to come.
- **Q&A sidebars:** These provide answers to some of the common questions related to each chapter topic.
- **Confidence Boosters:** Lack of confidence can hold nurses back from sharing their wealth of knowledge. These special sections are intended to build confidence and inspire.
- **Write Now!:** Exercises at the end of each chapter help students apply what they have learned.

The appendices include many additional resources:

- **Appendix A: Tips for Editing Checklist.** Students can use this to check their papers before submission.

- **Appendix B: Proofing Checklist.** This checklist should be completed immediately before submission.

- **Appendix C: Publishing Terminology.** Information here will help mitigate the intimidation many new authors feel when faced with publishing industry jargon.

- **Appendix D: Guidelines for Reporting Results.** Many journals require authors to follow established guidelines when reporting research or quality improvement projects. A table provides an overview of common guidelines and what they are used for.

- **Appendix E: Statistical Abbreviations.** This short list will help students use the correct abbreviations in their articles.

- **Appendix F: What Editors and Writers Want.** It's important to drive home that editors and writers are partners in any publishing endeavor.

- **Appendix G: Publishing Secrets From Editors.** This list provides honest insights from experienced editors.

This book can be used for a writing course or as a resource for courses in which students are expected to be able to use writing as a communication tool. It may be particularly helpful for students who wish to publish aspects of their doctor of nursing project.

This facilitator guide includes an overview of each chapter, followed by writing exercises that will help students apply what they have learned. Some of the exercises are in the book, while others are additional ones to provide the opportunity for more practice.

You might consider turning some of the exercises into group projects. For example, students could team up to create posters and present them to the rest of the students. All students could then vote for the best poster, with the winning team receiving a small prize. You also can encourage student interaction, for instance, by having students conduct a peer review of each other's papers.

PART I

A Primer on Writing and Publishing

1 Anatomy of Writing 2
Cynthia Saver

2 Finding, Refining, and Defining a Topic 3
Patricia Dwyer Schull and Cynthia Saver

3 How to Select and Query a Publication 4
Cynthia Saver

4 Finding and Documenting Sources 6
Leslie H. Nicoll

5 Organizing the Article 8
Kayla Little and Mary Alexander

6 Writing Skills Lab 9
Cynthia Saver

7 All About Graphics 11
Susanne J. Pavlovich-Danis

8 Submissions and Revisions 13
Patricia Gonce Morton and Tina M. Marrelli

9 Writing a Peer Review 14
Cindy L. Munro

10 Publishing for Global Authors 16
Susan Gennaro

11 Legal and Ethical Issues 17
Nancy J. Brent

12 Promoting Your Work 18
Timothy Landers and Stephanie J. Schulte

CHAPTER 1
Anatomy of Writing

This chapter introduces the analogy between writing and anatomy, so nurses can see that writing is more in line with their nursing knowledge than they might have originally thought. This analogy provides an overview of the entire writing process, which is then discussed in more detail in subsequent chapters. Key points include why it's important to write, how to overcome barriers, and how to write as part of a team. Chapter 1 serves as an overview of the publishing process, including a look at the roles on a publishing team.

Write Now!

1. In the space below, list three benefits you feel will come from writing an article. It might be personal satisfaction, a desire to learn more about a topic, or something else. The point is that it should be personal to you.

2. Write a few sentences about how you will carve out time in your schedule to write. Create action steps—for example, when will you set your first writing date in your calendar?

3. Consider this scenario: You are on a writing team of four people. The final draft of the article is done, but one person repeatedly ignores requests for input. What would you do? How could this situation have been avoided?

Comment

This is an opportunity to review the importance of the kickoff meeting and what it should include.

4. Here is another scenario: You want to write an article on strategies for improving nutrition in hospitalized patients. Who would be good writing team members for this topic?

5. Use the editing checklist in the Additional Resources section in the student workbook for your next writing project.

CHAPTER 2
Finding, Refining, and Defining a Topic

This chapter presents a series of questions students can use to identify a topic on which they would like to write. If they already have an idea, the questions can be used to evaluate the strength of the idea. A significant portion is dedicated to the process of narrowing a broad idea down to a more specific topic, with a special focus on mind mapping as a useful tool.

Write Now!

1. Use the right side of the table to answer the questions on the left.

Why should I write an article?	
Who will read my article?	
What interests me?	
What might interest others the most?	
What is happening at work or in my specialty?	
Which writing style should I use for a topic?	
What is the best timing for my article?	
Which publication is right for my article?	

2. Identify a topic of interest for your writing project. Use a mind map to narrow the focus of your idea. If you are stuck for a topic, consider how you would narrow the topic of "motivational interviewing." If you need more help with mind mapping, see https://www.mindtools.com/pages/article/newISS_01.htm.

3. Write a summary statement for your proposed article. Remember that this is one sentence that summarizes the entire article. Then see if it passes the "So what?" test by asking yourself why readers would care about the planned content. If you're not sure of a topic yet, write a summary statement for an article on pediatric delirium. Remember to be specific.

4. Create an outline for your topic idea.

Comment

This is an opportunity to note that an outline makes it easier to divide the work into blocks of time and is particularly helpful to keep a writing group focused.

CHAPTER 3
How to Select and Query a Publication

This chapter gives an overview of how to find possible publishing outlets and then explains what students should consider when deciding which to target. The "rights of medication administration" (which, although not a complete guide for administering medications, is an easy way to remember key points) is mirrored in this chapter's theme of the "rights of choosing a journal":

- Right audience
- Right numbers
- Right timing
- Right review process
- Right journal-level metrics

Additional topics covered in this chapter include open-access journals, alternative metrics, and predatory journals. The second part of the chapter discusses how to write an effective query letter.

Write Now!

1. In the space below, list three journals you feel would be a good fit for the topic you identified in Chapter 2's exercise. Then rank them in the order of best fit. (If you're not sure of your topic yet, list three journals suitable for the topic of palliative care in patients with end-stage heart failure.)

2. Evaluate at least one of your potential journals using the checklist from Think. Check. Submit. (http://thinkchecksubmit.org/journals).

3. Craft a query letter (email). You may find it helpful to use the template below as a guide.

Item to Include	Your Text
Name of editor, credentials, title	
Name of journal	
Brief statement of topic	
Why the topic would be of interest to the journal's readers	
Why you should be the one to write the article	
When you could submit the article	
Your name, credentials	
Your contact information (email and phone number)	

Comment
This is a good time to note that the publication's author guidelines often state whether the publication accepts queries.

4. Consider this scenario: You are two weeks from the deadline for your article when you receive a new assignment and realize you won't be able to complete the article. What would you do?

CHAPTER 4
Finding and Documenting Sources

This chapter explains how to find appropriate sources and how to cite and format those sources correctly. It also reviews types of style manuals. It includes an overview of databases, use of MeSH terms for searching, the ins and outs of bibliography database managers, and information on Digital Object Identifier (DOI) numbers. The chapter contains a short section on the difference between a student paper and an article for publication.

Write Now!

1. Conduct a search for the same terms in PubMed and Google Scholar and compare your results. (If you don't know what to search for, try "moral distress in nurses.") Which returned more results? What was the quality of the results?

2. Here is citation information for a fictitious article. Format the citation as a reference at the end of the article, first using APA style and then using AMA style.

   Author: Latoya M. Smith

   Title: "Effectiveness of a Computer-Based App in Improving Adherence with Medications in Older Adults with Chronic Obstructive Pulmonary Disease"

   Journal: *Journal of Pulmonary Nurses*

   Year: 2024

   Volume: 14

   Issue: 5

   Page numbers: 13–22

   DOI number: https://doi.org/10.xxxx

   APA style:

   AMA style:

Answer

APA style: Smith, L. M. (2024). Effectiveness of a computer-based app in improving adherence with medications in older adults with chronic obstructive pulmonary disease. *Journal of Pulmonary Nurses, 14*(5), 13–22. https://doi.org/10.xxxx

AMA style: Smith LM. Effectiveness of a computer-based app in improving adherence with medications in older adults with chronic obstructive pulmonary disease. *J Pulmon Nurs.* 2024;14(5):13-22. DOI: doi.org/10.xxxx

3. Download a free bibliography database manager such as Mendeley. Import some citations from the search you did in #1 into your library. Change the output style to APA, then AMA. Compare how the citations look.

4. Select three journals and identify the style of reference citation that each uses from looking at some articles. Then look at the information for authors for the journals. Do the guidelines specify which style manual to use for citations? Did you pick the right ones?

5. Watch the "PubMed: Overview" video at https://www.youtube.com/watch?v=1otz5qrUbxo, and then consider how PubMed and MEDLINE are different.

6. Improve your PubMed search skills by learning more about Medical Subject Headings (MeSH). The National Library of Medicine offers a free course at https://www.nlm.nih.gov/oet/ed/pubmed/mesh/index.html. For a quick overview, access the video "PubMed Subject Search: How It Works" at https://www.youtube.com/watch?v=6PhCRjQDfeI. For a more detailed video tutorial, access "How PubMed Works: Medical Subject Headings (MeSH)" at https://www.youtube.com/watch?v=xiHhFI_lG-U.

CHAPTER 5
Organizing the Article

This chapter introduces the basic format of an article (title, headings, beginning, middle, and end) and discusses abstracts, types of flow, and types of article structure (how to, case studies, IMRAD, disease process, chronological). It also presents templates for different types of articles (research, evidence-based practice, quality improvement, clinical, literature review, case study, nursing narratives). In addition, the chapter provides an overview of various reporting guidelines.

Write Now!

1. Choose three articles from two to three of your favorite nursing journals. List the name of the article and its type, such as research, evidence-based practice, quality improvement, clinical, literature review, or case study.

2. Pick a type of article you would like to write. Using a topic of your own choosing, summarize what you would include, using a template from the chapter.

3. Use the online tool from the EQUATOR Network (http://www.equator-network.org/toolkits/selecting-the-appropriate-reporting-guideline) to determine the most appropriate reporting guideline for a qualitative research report.

4. Compare the SQUIRE 2.0 (Standards for QUality Improvement Reporting Excellence) and the SRQR (Standards for Reporting Qualitative Research) guidelines. How are they similar and different?

CHAPTER 6
Writing Skills Lab

This chapter explains that effective writing meets the four Cs—clear, concise, correct, and compelling—and details how to achieve each "C." The basic writing principles will serve students well as they produce any type of written product for print or online. Topics include active/passive voice, parallelism, transitions, and the importance of bias-free writing.

Write Now!

1. Convert both of the following passive sentences into active sentences:

    Passive: Three main steps can be taken by nurses to improve pain management.

    Active: _____

    _____

    Passive: Phenomenological evidence of suffering and limitations wrought by pancreatic cancer that has been found in qualitative studies has resulted in an increased knowledge of living with pancreatic cancer.

    Active: _____

    _____

Possible answers

Active: Nurses can take three main steps to improve pain management.

Active: Qualitative studies have increased our knowledge of living with pancreatic cancer by providing phenomenological evidence of the suffering and limitations wrought by the disease.

2. Rework the list below so that each entry is parallel in structure.

    To start an IV, the nurse should:

    - Wear gloves.
    - The tourniquet should be tied a few centimeters above the location.
    - The patient should make a fist.
    - Find an appropriate vein.
    - Cleanse the skin with alcohol.
    - The alcohol should be allowed to dry completely.

Answer

To start an IV, the nurse should:

- Wear gloves.
- Tie the tourniquet a few centimeters above the location.
- Ask the patient to make a fist.
- Find an appropriate vein.
- Cleanse the skin with alcohol.
- Allow the alcohol to dry completely.

3. Identify the noun, verb, object, and qualifiers in the following sentences:

    The nurse finished her night shift on time.

    The trauma patient wakened to firm pressure.

Answers

The nurse finished her night shift on time. (nurse = noun, finished = verb, night = qualifier, shift = object, time = noun)

The trauma patient wakened to firm pressure. (trauma = qualifier, patient = noun, wakened = verb, firm = qualifier, pressure = noun)

4. Compare an article from *Nursing Research* to one from *American Nurse Journal*. How do they differ in tone, prevalence of passive/active voice, and use of references?
5. Pick an article from your favorite journal and identify active and passive sentences.

CHAPTER 7
All About Graphics

This chapter provides practical strategies for using graphics effectively. The student will learn about the various types of graphics that might be used, along with how to create strong graphics that best present the data or information. Other valuable sections include obtaining reprint permission, proper submission of graphics to a publication, and a table that helps writers select the right graphic based on purpose.

Write Now!

1. Which type of graphic or table would work best for each of the items below (more than one may be correct)?

Purpose	Graphic
Demographics of comparison groups	
Certification among the sample size of critical care nurses	
Comparison of health habits of patients with and without heart failure	
Process of early assessment and administration of t-PA for stroke	
New type of ventilator	

Answers
- Demographics of comparison groups (table or pie chart)
- Certification among the sample size of critical care nurses (pie chart)
- Comparison of health habits of patients with and without heart failure (bar chart)
- Process of early assessment and administration of t-PA for stroke (flowchart)
- New type of ventilator (photograph or illustration)

2. Pick a research article and a clinical article to review. Analyze the effectiveness of the graphics in each. How are graphics used in each type of article?

Comment
This can provide the opportunity to emphasize the value of graphics in conveying information.

3. In the space below, list three considerations for submitting an image to a journal.

Possible answers
Responses may include following the guidelines for submission, providing images of sufficient resolution, providing evidence of permission obtained for images under copyright, using the right format, and being sure all images are called out in the text.

CHAPTER 8
Submissions and Revisions

This chapter discusses the importance of following the author guidelines when submitting a manuscript and provides a submission checklist writers can use. Key points include the basics of the peer-review process and its role in achieving a quality publication. The latter part of the chapter acknowledges that criticism can at first be difficult to hear but assures the writer that constructive feedback is key to improving the manuscript. The focus is on moving beyond the initial reaction and on to the next steps—revision and resubmission of the manuscript. Types of requested revisions, how to format responses to reviewers, and what to do when reviewers disagree are all covered.

Write Now!

1. Identify a journal in which you are interested in publishing and review its submission guidelines and some past articles. Write a short paragraph as to the key points you'll want to keep in mind when submitting an article.

2. The next time you have to write something, use the proofing checklist in the Additional Resources section of the student workbook.

3. If you are a student, review the last paper you received comments on. Create a table that lists comments and your responses to those comments.

Comment	Response

CHAPTER 9
Writing a Peer Review

This chapter opens with a description of the peer-review process, including roles and responsibilities of peer reviewers, benefits of being a peer reviewer, how to become a reviewer, and types of peer review (double-anonymous, single-anonymous, and open review). The second part of the chapter explains how to write a peer review that will help authors improve their manuscript. Undergraduate students are unlikely to serve as peer reviewers; however, this chapter provides a helpful perspective for students who might find their own writing under peer review, as they learn what might be considered when evaluating an article.

Write Now!

1. List three topic areas where you feel you would have enough knowledge to serve as a peer reviewer for a colleague's article.

2. Consider contacting the editor of a journal that includes your topic area to offer your services as a peer reviewer.

3. Access the peer review process at https://www.elsevier.com/reviewers/what-is-peer-review. Write a short description of each type of review:

Review Type	Description
Single anonymous	
Double anonymous	
Open	

4. Ask a colleague if they would be willing to share an article they have written so that you can practice your peer-review skills. (Another option is to pick a published article in a journal you regularly read.) After you review it, write a short synopsis of the manuscript and your overall opinion. Summarize the major positive aspects. State the most important problems you've identified, how serious you think they are, and whether it's possible for the author to fix them. It may be helpful to first make notes on your thoughts as you review the following areas:

Content	Comments
Introduction	
Body	
Conclusion	
Graphics & tables	
References	

CHAPTER 10
Publishing for Global Authors

This chapter addresses the unique needs of authors in countries other than the United States. Readers learn how to determine if their work in one country serves a wider global audience. They will also find tips for writing in a second language and resources for non-native English-speaking authors.

Write Now!

1. Consider the challenges that authors for whom English is a second language face. If these authors cannot overcome these challenges, what will others lose as a result of not having access to their findings and insights?

2. Visit the *Journal of Nursing Scholarship* website and read one article from an author not from the United States. Summarize the article and its contribution to nursing.

3. The next time you have a project, consider involving an international partner to help you weigh global implications and possibly provide the opportunity to collaborate.

Comment

This is a good place to reinforce that if global authors don't have opportunities to publish, knowledge that could help patients may not be widely disseminated.

CHAPTER 11
Legal and Ethical Issues

This chapter first reviews the legal issues related to publishing, such as copyright, permissions, and fair use of content. The second half of the chapter discusses ethics of publishing, including authorship, conflicts of interest, confidentiality, privacy, and research misconduct. Readers can find legal information worrisome, so it helps to reassure them that following good publication practices will help avert potential problems.

Write Now!

1. You would like to reproduce Figure 3.1, which shows a model of how to analyze delirium from the *Journal of Cognitive Dysfunction*. The model was on page 15 of an article written by T. Monk and G. Christie, which appeared in volume 6, issue 5, pages 14–20. You wish to use the model in your upcoming article in assessment of delirium in long-term care patients. Write a permission letter to the publisher (Publisher Group A) for the journal. (All journal information is fictitious.)

2. Visit the *Journal of Nursing Education* website at https://www.healio.com/nursing/journals/jne/submit-an-article and review its guidelines for submitting an article. Summarize the section related to human subjects protection.

3. Compare and contrast other requirements for publishing in nursing journals for consistency and differences.

4. Pretend you want to publish an article you wrote under a Creative Commons license. Use the Creative Commons Tool to find the recommended type of license based on your preferences: https://chooser-beta.creativecommons.org.

5. Your article has been accepted for publication by a nursing journal. The topic is one you wrote a student paper on, but the article is significantly different. Does the instructor who graded the paper and gave you feedback qualify for authorship? Why or why not?

Comment

Here is where you can emphasize authorship criteria and how authorship differs from acknowledgments. You may also want to take this time to review the problems with using generative artificial intelligence (AI) and note that use of any AI must be disclosed to the publication upon submission.

CHAPTER 12
Promoting Your Work

This chapter emphasizes the importance of marketing your work if you want to be effective in disseminating information. Too often, nurses don't think about marketing until later in their careers, but starting early is best. Strategies covered in the chapter include picking the right keywords and using them effectively, social media and academia social networking sites, in-person networking, author-level metrics, and working with media outlets. This chapter would also be helpful for a professional development course.

Write Now!

1. Identify two or three target audiences who might be interested in the topics you most like to write about, and then describe the top two points of interest for each group.

2. Pick an article from a journal, and then practice writing social media messages for X, Facebook, and Instagram that promote the article.

3. If you don't have one already, create a free LinkedIn profile. If you have started your research journey, create an Open Researcher and Contributor ID (ORCID) account.

4. Make a list of potential magazines or news outlets that would be interested in your topic.

5. Write a plain language summary of a review of your choosing. Aim to write it so that a person without any background in healthcare can understand it. What was the experience of translating what you learned from the review into a summary that a "lay" knowledge user can understand?

Comment

Many authors neglect to promote their work, so it's a good idea to provide sufficient practice time with the different strategies.

At the end of Part I, the workbook has the following flowchart of the publishing process that can be used as a reference.

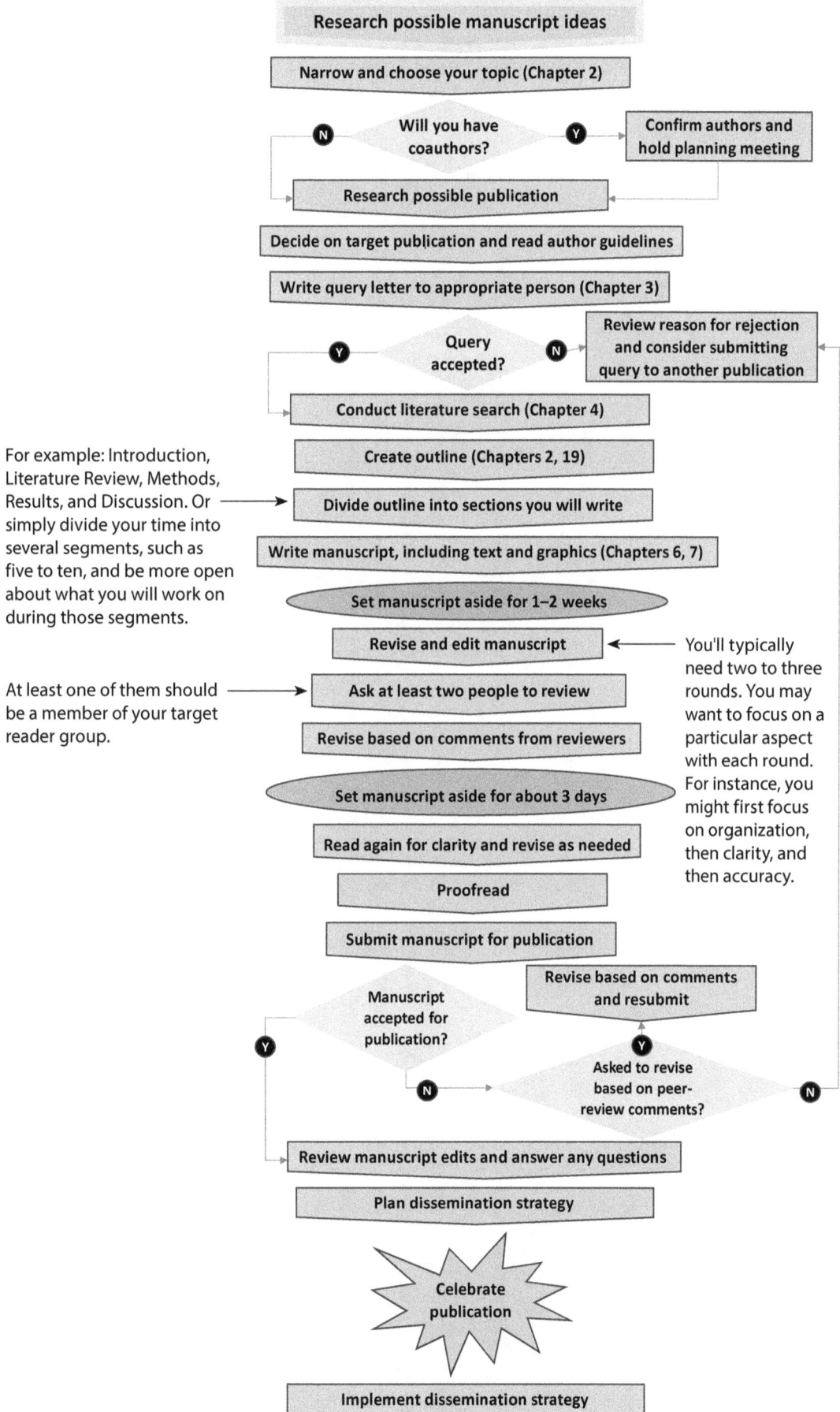

PART II

Tips for Writing Different Types of Articles

13 Writing the Clinical Article 22
Cheryl L. Mee and Fidelindo Lim

14 Writing the Research Report 23
Patricia Gonce Morton

15 Writing the Review Article 24
Lisa Hopp

16 Reporting the Quality Improvement or Evidence-Based Practice Project 25
Jo Rycroft-Malone and Christopher Burton

17 Writing for Presentations 27
Rose O. Sherman

18 From Student Project or Dissertation to Publication 28
Deborah Lindell and Lorraine Steefel

19 Writing a Continuing Professional Development Activity 29
Nadine Salmon

20 Writing the Nursing Narrative 30
Marianne Ditomassi

21 Think Outside the Journal: Alternative Publication Options 32
Demetrius J. Porche

22 Writing a Book or Book Chapter 33
Sandra M. Nettina

23 Writing for a General Audience 34
Pamela J. Haylock

CHAPTER 13
Writing the Clinical Article

This chapter covers one of the most common types of articles nurses write—the clinical article. It differentiates a clinical article from a scholarly one and takes readers through a stepped approach to writing a clinical article: develop a topic and focus, select a journal for publication, send a query email, choose an appropriate format, gather information, prepare to write, write using authoritative and active voice, edit the manuscript, submit, and revise as needed based on peer-review comments.

Write Now!

1. List two possible ideas for a clinical article. Look for a prototype format(s) (e.g., case study, how to, disease state) that fits your topic.

2. Write a title for one of the topics. Be sure the title is enticing to readers. Also, try to improve on this title: "Compassion Fatigue."

3. Write a case study article on a topic of your choosing. If you are having trouble choosing a topic, consider this option: a patient who is newly diagnosed with diabetes.

4. Identify the subheads in the chapter or in a published clinical article.

5. Find the regular departments or columns in one or two clinical journals. Consider what topic you could write about that would fit one of them. (Review the author guidelines.)

Comment

This is a good place to reinforce that departments are a good avenue for breaking into writing.

CHAPTER 14
Writing the Research Report

This chapter is vital for those pursuing research as part of their career path because it explains in detail how to write a research report. It reviews each section of a typical report (abstract, introduction, methods, results, and discussion) and teaches the elements of crafting a strong abstract. The chapter covers quantitative, qualitative, and mixed-methods studies and contains a table that compares the three.

Write Now!

1. Read a published article without reviewing the abstract. Then use the OJISH mnemonic to write an abstract for the article and compare it to the published abstract. Use the table below to record your initial thoughts.

Step	Notes
Outline a pressing problem in the field.	
Justify a new study with a gap in the literature.	
Introduce the purpose of the proposed or present study.	
Summarize the methodology.	
Highlight the major findings.	

2. Review the abstract from the study by Zangaro and colleagues (2023) included in the chapter, and then formulate one or two research questions and several hypotheses you may wish to test if you were doing this study. Next, read the entire article and see if any of your questions/hypotheses match those of the authors.

3. Read the results section of two research articles and note how the authors have used tables and figures to supplement the article. Critique the two articles in how well they presented their results and the extent to which tables and figures helped you understand what the authors were trying to convey. What would you do differently?

4. Write the data analysis section for an article reporting the results of a qualitative study of nurses' reactions when caring for patients in the middle of a pandemic. Refer to the chapter for guidelines as to what you should include.

CHAPTER 15
Writing the Review Article

This chapter discusses the value of review articles and provides guidance for writing the most common types—systematic (both quantitative and qualitative), scoping, and integrative. Two tables are particularly valuable: one compares the three review types discussed in the chapter and the other presents additional types of review articles.

Write Now!

1. Find an example of a systematic review, a scoping review, and an integrative review. Compare them carefully to differentiate their purposes, methods, findings, and conclusions.

2. Read a published systematic review without reading the abstract. Then, write one following the elements of a systematic review. Did you find similar conclusions as the investigators who published the review?

3. Find an appraisal tool for one type of review (e.g., find the CASP tool for systematic reviews). Read the review and identify its strengths and weakness.

4. Use the PICO (P = population, I = intervention, C = comparator, O = outcome) method to write a question for a systematic review.

CHAPTER 16
Reporting the Quality Improvement or Evidence-Based Practice Project

This chapter guides authors through the process of writing articles about quality improvement (QI) or evidence-based practice (EBP) projects. It answers common questions about these two types of projects, such as how they differ from research studies and who target readers might be. Next, the chapter reviews how to write these articles, including use of the SQUIRE guidelines.

Write Now!

1. Think about a QI or EBP project that you have either led or been involved in. Write an outline for an article, including subheadings and sample text for each section. Consider how you might involve other relevant stakeholders in this planning process.

2. Pick a QI or EBP article from a journal and analyze it using the framework discussed in the chapter. How would you improve the article? The table below may be helpful.

Element	Your Comments
Title (Does it clearly convey what the article is about?)	
Abstract (Does it provide background, methods, findings, and conclusions?)	
Introduction (Does it explain why the project was done?)	
Methods (Does it clearly describe what was done, by whom, and where? Does it address ethical considerations?)	
Results (Does it describe what changes were made?)	
Discussion (Does it provide a useful overview?)	
Conclusion and implications (Does it consider implications and wider applicability?)	

3. Think about a QI project you have been involved in, and note what categories the interventions fell into using the table below as a guide.

Types of Interventions	Examples	My Project
Professional	Distribution of educational materials, local consensus processes, audit and feedback, reminders	
Financial	Fee-for-service, incentives	
Organizational	Revision of professional roles, skill mix change, patient involvement, changing documentation systems	
Regulatory	Management of patient complaints, peer review	

Comment

Editors frequently receive articles identified by the author as research when they are really EBP or QI projects, so it's a good idea to review the differences.

CHAPTER 17
Writing for Presentations

This chapter discusses writing an abstract for a talk or poster presentation. Key topics include how to review the call for abstracts. A sample reviewer evaluation form is provided so the reader can see what reviewers look for, and a case study presents the entire process. The chapter also gives readers tips for creating effective posters and encourages presenters to write an article based on their talk or poster.

Write Now!

1. Pick one of the calls for abstracts at https://www.sigmanursing.org/connect-engage/meetings-events/calls-for-abstracts. Download the guidelines and write a submission.

2. Use the guidelines in the chapter and at https://guides.lib.unc.edu/posters/pptwindows2016 to create a poster; the data can be fictitious.

3. List three possible titles for your poster from #2 and describe why you chose the one you did.

4. Visit the website of a professional organization in your specialty area and look for the date of the next conference and when the call for abstracts will be posted. Create a timeline for submitting an abstract for a poster or podium presentation.

CHAPTER 18
From Student Project or Dissertation to Publication

This chapter helps students understand that a school assignment must be reworked before it can be published and provides a process for doing so. It then goes into more detail about how to rework academic work to create published articles. This chapter is a must-read for any student considering publishing work that started as a school presentation or paper.

Write Now!

1. Choose one assignment that you are passionate about or did well on and research journals and magazines that would be appropriate for an article related to your work.

2. Find out your school's requirements related to sharing work in databases.

3. Create a short outline for a possible article based on a paper you completed for a school project.

4. Download (and use) the School Paper to Manuscript Student Checklist at https://onlinelibrary.wiley.com/pb-assets/assets/17504910/Checklist%20pdfs/6-School-Paper-to-Manuscript-Student-Checklist-1599562514443.pdf.

Comment

The checklist is a useful tool for converting academic work.

CHAPTER 19
Writing a Continuing Professional Development Activity

This chapter discusses how to write an effective nursing continuing professional development (NCPD) or an interprofessional continuing education (IPCE) learning activity, including understanding the target audience; choosing a topic; writing goals, objectives, and outcome statements; creating an outline; writing the content; and developing the post-test. While this chapter is geared more toward practicing nurses, it can be valuable for undergraduate students as a guide to help make them more informed CE program consumers.

Write Now!

1. State the goal of an educational activity you would like to write.

2. Write two learning objectives related to the goal. For each one, note the level of learning the objective will measure, based on Bloom's taxonomy. The table below may be helpful.

Level of Learning	Type of Learning	Verbs
Knowledge	Memorization and regurgitation	Define, identify, list, repeat, name, relate
Comprehension	Understanding and interpretation	Discuss, describe, report, explain, review, summarize
Application	Use of information in new situation	Translate, apply, interpret, demonstrate
Analysis	Breakup of the whole into parts	Distinguish, compare showing relationships, contrast, differentiate
Synthesis	Combination of elements, forming new structure	Formulate, prepare, design, assemble, plan
Evaluation	Situation assessment, based on criteria	Assess, compute, revise, measure, evaluate

3. Now, instead of objectives, write two outcome statements. Remember to focus on what learners are expected to do after completing the activity. (After completing this program, the learner will be able to...)

4. Pick an NCPD program from a journal and write four post-test questions for it. If you can, compare what you wrote to the published questions.

CHAPTER 20
Writing the Nursing Narrative

This chapter explains the value of narratives and provides examples of each type—advocacy, error, interdisciplinary teamwork, reflection, resilience, and skill acquisition. The examples are from real nurses, and each one includes commentary. The chapter then delves into how to write an effective narrative and concludes with a discussion on getting nursing narratives published. The chapter can be used to reinforce to students that narratives may be required for clinical advancement, so it's important to gain expertise with this type of writing.

Write Now!

1. Write a narrative. Visualize a patient you cared for or a situation that has stayed with you. Recall what you saw, heard, smelled, and felt. Write the experience as you remember it. Include dialogue and the thoughts and feelings you had at the time. (Be sure to change the patient's name and any other identifying information to protect privacy and confidentiality.) The table below may help you get started.

Information to Include	Your Notes
Name, title, unit, and length of time in practice	
A detailed description of what happened	
Why this situation is important to you	
What your concerns were at the time	
What you were thinking about as it was taking place	
What you were feeling during and after the situation	
What, if anything, stood out to you	

2. Keep a journal for one week to help you identify future ideas for narratives.

3. Use a mobile device or tape recorder to tell a story to yourself, or speak to a trusted colleague about a patient you cared for. Tell it quickly, without judgment or editing yourself. Then listen to the story for key points you might include in a narrative.

4. Review narratives published in *Caring Headlines* (https://www.mghpcs.org/caring/caring-previous.shtml), a publication of Massachusetts General Hospital, and identify their types.

CHAPTER 21
Think Outside the Journal: Alternative Publication Avenues

This chapter covers publishing options that don't immediately come to mind (such as letters to the editor, editorials, columns, books reviews, newsletters, and blogs) but which can be writing opportunities for nurses. Readers learn about these options and strategies for writing them. These small writing projects may seem more achievable for novice authors.

Write Now!

1. Write a letter (email) to the editor and submit it. Read any guidelines before you write.

2. Review your professional association's, school's, or hospital's newsletter. Identify the three main areas that are the focus. What could you contribute as an article in one of these areas?

3. Write a blog on a nursing topic you feel passionate about.

4. Select a journal you read routinely. Does the journal publish columns? If so, read the author guidelines for writing a column. Review the last two years of the journal for relevant and "hot" topics not covered. Contact the editor to see if there is interest in your topic.

CHAPTER 22
Writing a Book or Book Chapter

This chapter takes authors from idea to published book. It includes preparation such as targeting a publisher, crafting a successful proposal, developing a table of contents, using a template for contributors' content, and creating a sample chapter. It covers the advantages and challenges of working with contributors as well as helpful pointers for choosing contributors. The chapter also discusses legal considerations (such as contracts), creating a schedule, and the various parts of the book.

Write Now!

1. Compare the table of contents from three different books to identify different formats. Analyze how well the table of contents reflects the book's stated purpose and title.

2. Think of an idea for a book. Using the Sigma Theta Tau International proposal format below, make notes on how you would accomplish each step.

Information	Your Notes
Working title	
Name of the authors, editors, and any contributors already identified	
Description of topic and how the book uniquely addresses a need in the market	
Primary audience	
Number of chapters and projected word count	
Special features	
Time frame	
Goals for writing this book	
Competitive works	
Table of contents	

Comment

This is more advanced content, so it might be a good opportunity to use the team approach to developing the outline of a proposal.

CHAPTER 23
Writing for a General Audience

This chapter discusses how to write for laypeople in need of healthcare information. It describes principles of writing for a general audience, such as delivering a clear and compelling message, and factors important to consider, such as literacy, reading level, and cultural sensitivity. The chapter revisits the letter to the editor, this time for a general publication, and can be used to emphasize to students that nurses are well positioned to deliver health-related information to the public.

Write Now!

1. Pick a health-related article on the website of a consumer publication outlet and evaluate it using the checklist for plain language (https://www.plainlanguage.gov/resources/checklists/web-checklist). Rate each item on a 3-point scale, with 3 being completely meeting the criterion.

    - Less is more! Be concise.
    - Break documents into separate topics.
    - Use even shorter paragraphs than on paper.
    - Use short lists and bullets to organize information.
    - Use even more lists than on paper.
    - Use even more headings with less under each heading (questions often make great headings).
    - Present each topic or point separately and use descriptive section headings.
    - Keep the information on each page to no more than two levels.
    - Make liberal use of white space so pages are easy to scan.
    - Write (especially page titles) using the same words your readers would use when doing a web search for the info.
    - Don't assume your readers have knowledge of the subject or have read related pages on your site. Clearly explain things so each page can stand on its own.
    - Never use "click here" as a link. Link language should describe what your reader will get if they click the link.
    - Eliminate unnecessary words.

2. Write a paragraph designed for the public, and then test its readability level using the tool in your word-processing program.

3. Pick two or three paragraphs from a published journal article and rewrite them for a general audience.

Comment
It may be helpful to mention that some journals require authors to develop plain language summaries.

Duty to Disseminate

I hope that this guide will help you as you encourage your students to write. I believe nurses have a professional duty to disseminate their knowledge and expertise—sharing valuable information promotes excellence in practice and improves the lives of our patients. Establishing writing expectations during the student years helps establish a career-long writing habit.

Above all, the contributors and I salute you for all your hard work in teaching future nurses and nurses who wish to advance in their careers.

Cynthia Saver, MS, RN
Editor
Anatomy of Writing for Publication for Nurses, Fifth Edition